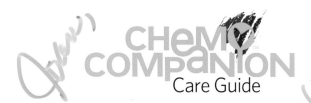

CHEMO COMPANION
Care Guide

Written by

Jean E. Sprengel, MD

with

Lanette Sprengel Mohr

Foreword By
Best-Selling Author and Cancer Survivor
Dr. Benjamin S. Carson Sr.

SPRENGEL & SONS
P.O. Box 8141
Redlands, CA 92375
chemocompanioncareguide@gmail.com

Publisher's note: The information in this book is not in-
tended as a substitute for professional medical advice and
treatment. Your own doctor is the best person to advise you
regarding your own personal situation. As such, no ex-
pressed or implied guarantee can be given nor liability taken.

Dedicated to my sister Kaye,
my very best friend.

CONTENTS

A ROAD WELL-TRAVELED - *Foreword* 6

A FELLOW TRAVELER - *Introduction* 8

SETTING THE COURSE – *Preparing for Chemo*

SAY AHHH! 12
Dental Care

GOTCHA COVERED 19
Head Coverings

EXERCISE YOUR OPTIONS 15
IV Access

IT'S IN THE BAG 23
Chemo Bag

LET'S GET STARTED – *Chemo DAY*

DAY ONE 27
What to Expect

THE ROAD AHEAD – *Side Effects of Chemo*

TAKE IT EASY 31
Fatigue

LOSING IT 36
Your Hair, That Is

FOGGED IN 33
Chemo Brain

KEEP IT DOWN 39
Nausea and Vomiting

OUCH! 35
Pain

ON THE RUN 40
Intestinal Problems

THE ROAD AHEAD *(cont.)*

CULINARY CHALLENGE 44
Changes in Appetite

UP, UP AND AWAY 57
Fluid Retention

INSIDE OUT 47
Sore Mouth, Gums, and Throat

JUST ADD WATER 59
Kidney and Bladder Irritation

SCALES TO NAILS 49
Skin and Nail Problems

STAY IN TOUCH 61
Sex and Reproduction

NICE N' EASY 52
Nerve and Muscle Problems

LOOK AGAIN 64
Changes in Blood Cell Count

LOOKIN' GOOD 55
Eye and Vision Changes

CONSTANT COMPANION – *A Natural High!*

LAUGHTER 71
The Best Medicine

TRAVEL TIPS - *Quotes From Chemo Graduates* 74

ENTOURAGE - *Acknowledgments* 76

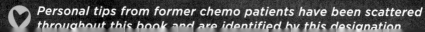

Personal tips from former chemo patients have been scattered throughout this book and are identified by this designation.

A Road Well-Traveled
Foreword

When I was an intern at Johns Hopkins, I remember being very impressed by the titles of some of the patients I saw being treated there. They were CEOs of major companies, presidents of large organizations and crown princes of various countries—all dying of some malignant disease. Witnessing this helped me really appreciate how important life is, as I realized that each of these very rich and powerful people would gladly give up every penny and title they had for a clean bill of health.

Even though you have been diagnosed with cancer, your diagnosis has come at a time of tremendous breakthroughs in various cancer treatments. More is known today about what works and what doesn't in terms of maximizing comfort during the treatment phase than ever before. You will learn about all this and more in this booklet.

One of the biggest challenges cancer patients face is their fear. I remember vividly the day I learned I had a very aggressive form of prostate cancer. It very quickly put things into perspective for me, but at the same time, my biggest fear was that I would be leaving my loved ones behind. Fear can have very detrimental effects on the balance of many bodily functions. If cancer patients are plagued by fears and anxieties their bodily functions can and most likely will continue to deteriorate. That is why I am delighted with this companion booklet, which addresses many of the most common fears in an understandable, light-hearted manner. I only wish I would have had something like this at the time of my diagnosis.

Whether you are a recently diagnosed cancer patient or a family member or friend of someone recently diagnosed, there is no question that difficult times lay ahead. Just know you will not have to travel through those hard times alone. Many have traveled the road before you and many are traveling alongside you right now. My hope is that this pocket companion will be an additional source of comfort and information for you to use during your time of need. May God bless you and bring you peace and health in the long run.

Benjamin S. Carson Sr., MD
Professor and Director of Pediatric Neurosurgery
Johns Hopkins Children's Center

*Dr. Carson is also a Medal of Freedom Recipient and
the President and Co-Founder of Carson Scholars Fund*

A Fellow Traveler
Introduction

In 1996 my sister, Kaye, was diagnosed with breast cancer. Although initially frightened, we were a little relieved to learn she had ductal carcinoma in situ (DCIS), as DCIS is considered to be the mildest form of breast cancer. Being the athlete she is, Kaye had her mastectomy and was windsurfing two weeks later.

Around Christmas of 2007 she was diagnosed with a recurrence of the cancer. This time it had spread to her liver, which meant chemotherapy and the very real threat of losing my best friend.

I have been a practicing physician for more than 25 years but as an anesthesiologist, not an oncologist. I knew that I had to trust her oncologist to take care of her cancer and to focus on what I could do best—to take care of her as a person.

I searched the Internet and spent hours talking to everyone I knew who had personal experience with chemo. I was determined that Kaye would be prepared and ready to meet this threat head-on, armed with all the information and tools she would need. My mission was to make things easier and more comfortable for her as she faced the greatest challenge of her life.

The original copy of the book you are holding is what I wrote for my sister. In addition to this Chemo Companion, I created a "chemo bag," stuffed with all the necessities and treats she would need. With this book as her guide and her barf bucket by her side, she was poised to make this journey as gracefully as possible.

This little book doesn't have all the answers, so please use a book specific to your type of cancer and chemo as a reference or make sure you have easy access to the Internet. While this companion book does not take the place of talking to your health care providers, it is my fervent hope that it will help you as you prepare for the road ahead.

Best wishes on your journey,

Jean E. Sprengel, M.D.

Jean E. Sprengel, MD

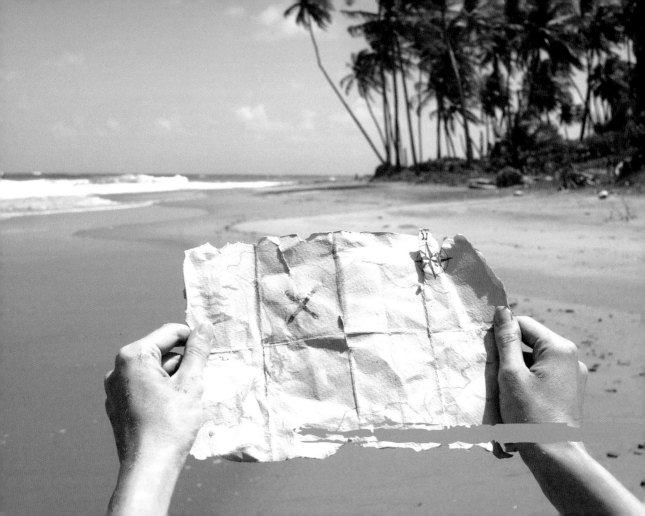

SETTING THE COURSE
PREPARING FOR CHEMO

The decision has been made. Chemotherapy. It may be a relief to have that part behind you, but you're probably pretty nervous about what comes next. On the following pages you will find a few things to consider before you begin.

SAY AHHH!
Dental Care 12

EXERCISE YOUR OPTIONS
IV Access 15

GOTCHA COVERED
Head Coverings 19

IT'S IN THE BAG
Chemo Bag 23

SAY AHHH!
DENTAL CARE

You may think that the chemo drugs will head straight for your cancer but the truth is, they detour throughout your body, including your mouth. To prevent damage to your teeth, make sure they are clean and free from disease *before* starting chemo. Make an appointment to see your dentist today and be sure to mention your upcoming chemo treatments.

A common side effect of chemo is a dry mouth, caused by the reduction of saliva. This causes tooth decay because saliva is needed to neutralize acids from food and dental plaque. Since you are more susceptible to infection during chemo, any problem areas need prompt attention by your dentist.

The following list includes guidelines for proper oral care:

- Have a dental checkup every 1–3 months.
- Ask your dentist about fluoride treatments.
- Brush and floss after every meal, snack and before bedtime.
- Use a soft toothbrush and soak it in water to soften it before brushing.
- Make sure your mouthwash DOES NOT contain alcohol.
- Help keep your mouth moist by using artificial saliva.
- Drink lots of fluorinated water.
- If you wear dentures, your mouth's dryness may cause them to lose their proper fit. Visit your dentist if this becomes a problem.
- Avoid eating acidic, spicy and hot foods.
- Avoid soft drinks—they are acidic.

Do you snore? People who snore while sleeping or breathe through their mouths are particularly susceptible to a dry mouth. If this describes you, keep water and/or artificial saliva at your bedside to use when you wake during the night.

Note: BIOTENE® brand products specifically address dry mouth issues.

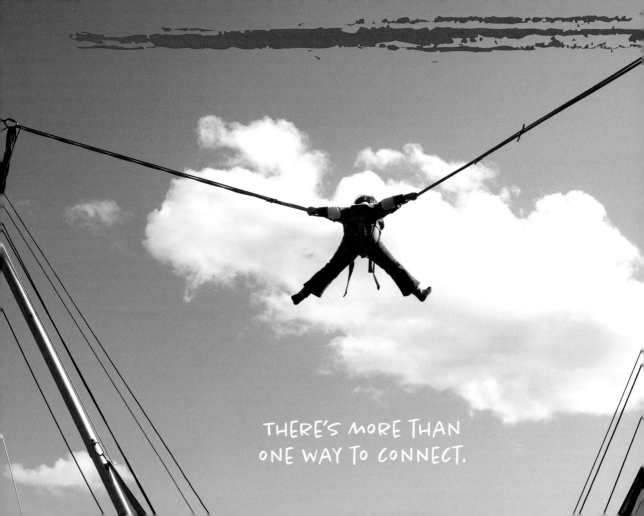

THERE'S MORE THAN
ONE WAY TO CONNECT.

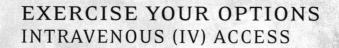

EXERCISE YOUR OPTIONS
INTRAVENOUS (IV) ACCESS

Depending on the type of medication you receive and the length of your chemo treatment, you may want to ask your doctor if a more permanent intravenous (IV) access device is right for you. Why? When the veins in your arms are used repeatedly, they eventually get hard and become unusable, requiring multiple attempts to start an IV.

Some options to consider:

A **portacath** is an intravenous access line that goes into a vein in the chest, with the entrance just below your collarbone or on the upper arm. It requires a small surgery to insert, but this can often be done under local anesthesia with some sedation, or at the same time as another surgery you may need for your cancer.

The portacath is hidden under the skin and only a small lump can be seen and felt. With a portacath in place, the nurses simply insert a needle into the port instead of searching for a vein, making insertion much easier and more comfortable.

A **peripherally inserted central catheter**, or a **PICC** line, is like a regular IV started in the arm. During a simple procedure, a nurse inserts a long, thin catheter into a vein in the arm and threads it until it reaches a large vein just above the heart. Medication is connected to this tubing, instead of poking you with needles. This kind of IV cannot be left in as long as a portacath because there is a higher risk of infection, but this may be an ideal option for a shorter course of treatment.

Hickman and *Broviac* **catheters** are two other options that are similar to a portacath. However, their access ports are not buried under the skin, so from a patient's perspective, they behave more like a PICC line and share advantages and disadvantages with both.

Don't worry about making this decision on your own. Talk with your oncologist about all your options so they can help you decide which one is best for you and your specific treatment.

LET YOUR FRIENDS KNOW THAT IT'S OK TO TALK ABOUT YOUR CANCER. DON'T LET IT BE THE ELEPHANT IN THE ROOM THAT NO ONE MENTIONS. PEOPLE DON'T KNOW WHAT TO SAY, SO GIVE THEM PERMISSION TO DO THEIR BEST.

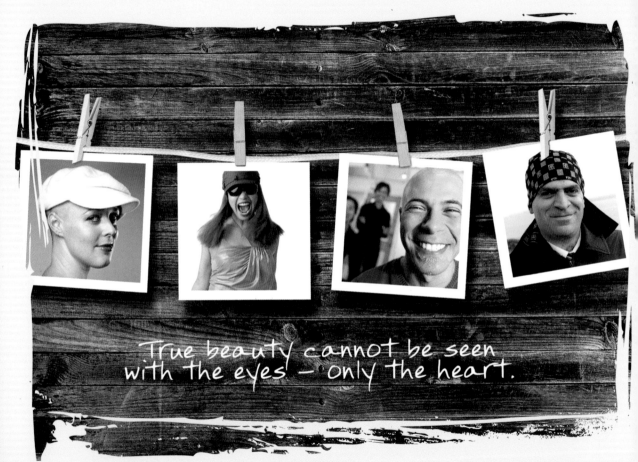

True beauty cannot be seen
with the eyes — only the heart.

Gotcha Covered
Head Coverings

When people hear "chemotherapy," most think "hair loss." The good news is that not everyone loses their hair with chemo. If you do— there are lots of options. Your doctor and nurses can tell you if hair loss is one of the expected side effects of *your* specific treatment. If it is, consider the options available to deal with this loss *before* it starts.

Get creative
Show off your individual style and have some fun by asking friends and family to pick out a hat for you. Everyone looks great in baseball caps and don't forget about scarves and beanies. And if you're brave enough—go bald! Just remember that your head *will* get cold, especially at night.

"Go shopping for hats and wigs with the most honest friend you know."

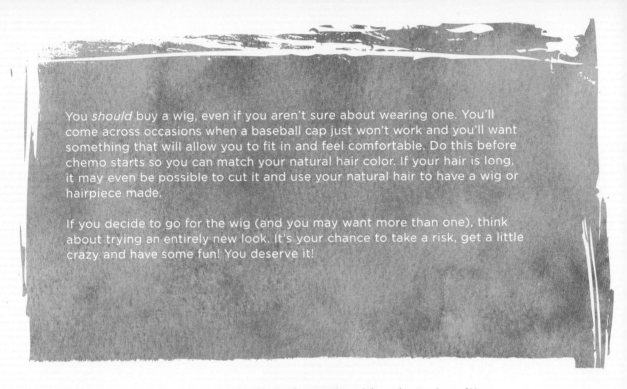

You *should* buy a wig, even if you aren't sure about wearing one. You'll come across occasions when a baseball cap just won't work and you'll want something that will allow you to fit in and feel comfortable. Do this before chemo starts so you can match your natural hair color. If your hair is long, it may even be possible to cut it and use your natural hair to have a wig or hairpiece made.

If you decide to go for the wig (and you may want more than one), think about trying an entirely new look. It's your chance to take a risk, get a little crazy and have some fun! You deserve it!

Some insurance companies will pay for a wig with a doctor's written prescription for a "cranial prosthesis." If not, ask your accountant about deducting the cost of the wig as a medical expense on your income tax.

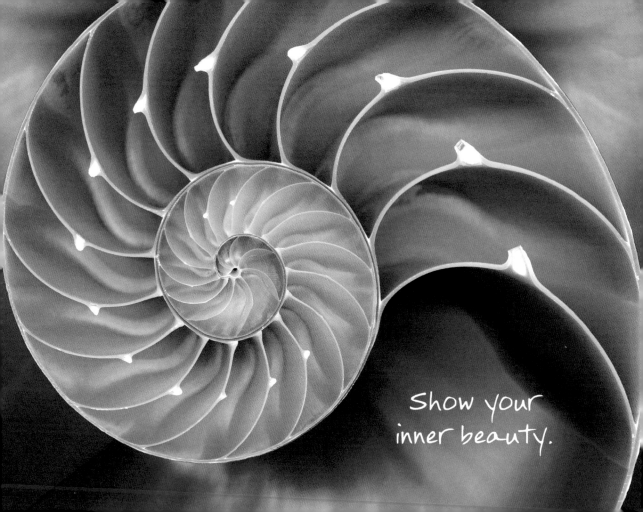

Show your
inner beauty.

SAVE THE DATE!
CALL YOUR FRIEND WITH
THE DATE FOR YOUR
FIRST DAY OF CHEMO.

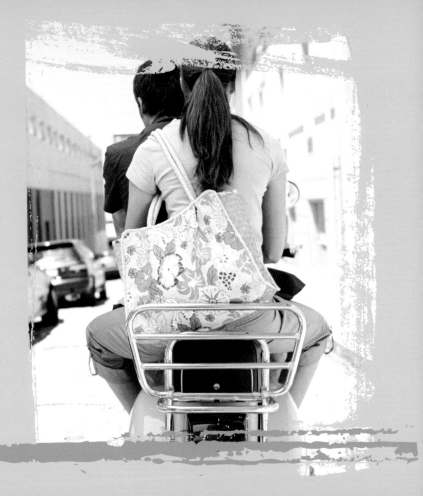

IT'S IN THE BAG
CHEMO BAG

A great way to help you manage your treatment is by creating a bag of personal things that will help keep you comfortable during your chemo days. Here are some suggestions to get you started:

- A water bottle. It's important to KEEP HYDRATED!
- Saltine crackers to fight the metallic taste chemo can cause
- Regular or ginger mints to calm an upset stomach
- Lip balm or lip gloss
- Blanket, socks and a sweater. Chemo units can get cold!
- A small pillow or neck roll
- A personal music player
- A book, crossword puzzles or Sudoku puzzles
- DVDs—some facilities have TVs, others have DVD players
- A close friend or family member. (Just keep in mind they might not actually fit in the bag!)

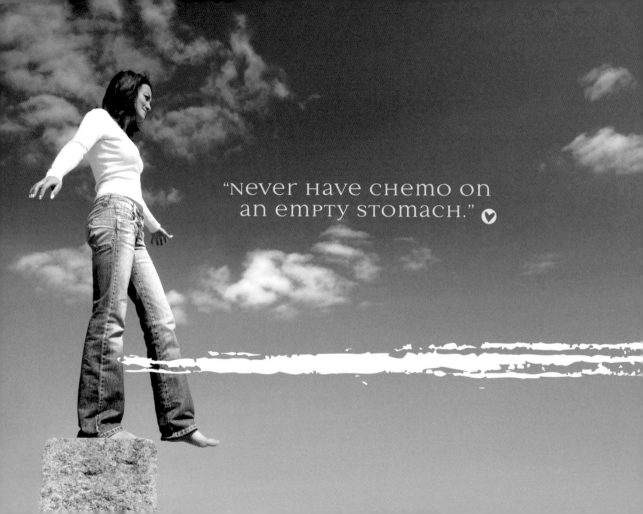

"never have chemo on
an empty stomach."

LET'S GET STARTED
CHEMO DAY

Beginning your chemo day with a light breakfast will help your stomach tolerate the effects of the chemo drugs. Choose comfortable clothing with a loose-fitting waist and don't forget your "chemo bag." Your nurses can tell you ahead of time how long your treatment will take to help you plan your day.

DAY ONE
What to Expect 27

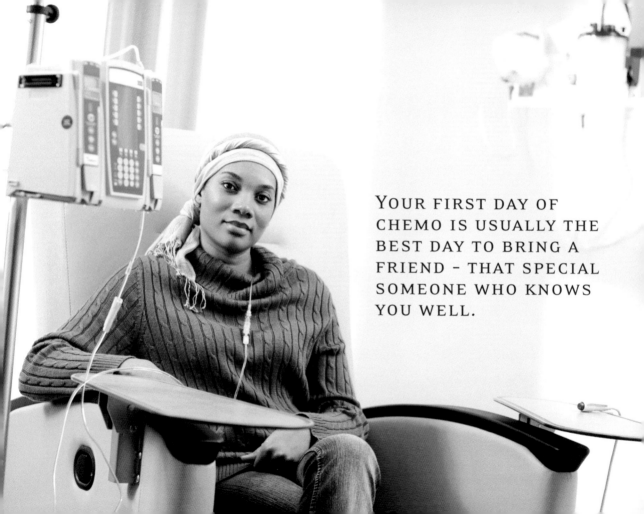

YOUR FIRST DAY OF
CHEMO IS USUALLY THE
BEST DAY TO BRING A
FRIEND – THAT SPECIAL
SOMEONE WHO KNOWS
YOU WELL.

DAY ONE
WHAT TO EXPECT

Most chemotherapy centers have a large room with lots of reclining chairs and often each chair will have its own TV and/or DVD player to entertain you. Once you are comfortably settled, a nurse will begin your treatment with premeds, including things like steroids and anti-nausea medicines, followed by the chemo drugs. This is not a painful or uncomfortable experience. The fact is, boredom is more likely to be a problem. When the chemo drugs are completed, the nurse will run normal saline through the IV to make sure that your veins are cleared of the chemo drugs. This will help to keep them soft for your next treatment.

When the nausea kicks in
You're probably expecting your first dose of chemo to include a stomach ache and nausea. Rest easy this round. Typically, nausea doesn't start until later that night or the following day. For most patients, the worst day tends to be the third day following treatment. Once you make it past this point, you'll start to feel better.

THE ROAD AHEAD
SIDE EFFECTS OF CHEMO

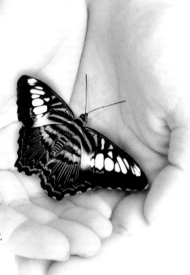

There are many different chemotherapy protocols used by oncologists and they change continually as new drugs are developed in the fight against cancer. The side effects that you experience will be determined by which drugs you take and whether they are in IV or pill form. Ask your doctor which of these side effects you are most likely to encounter. You will then be able to better prepare for the effects of *your* treatment.

"Write on a calendar how you are feeling every day. You will soon see patterns to help predict how you will react and you will know what to report to your doctor."

SIDE EFFECTS

TAKE IT EASY
Fatigue 31

FOGGED IN
Chemo Brain 33

OUCH!
Pain 35

LOSING IT
Your Hair, That Is 36

KEEP IT DOWN
Nausea and Vomiting 39

ON THE RUN
Intestinal Problems 40

CULINARY CHALLENGE
Changes in Appetite 44

INSIDE OUT
Sore Mouth, Gums, and Throat 47

SCALES TO NAILS
Skin and Nail Problems 49

NICE N' EASY
Nerve and Muscle Problems 52

LOOKIN' GOOD
Eye and Vision Changes 55

UP, UP AND AWAY
Fluid Retention 57

JUST ADD WATER
Kidney and Bladder Irritation 59

STAY IN TOUCH
Sex and Reproduction 61

LOOK AGAIN
Changes in Blood Cell Count 64

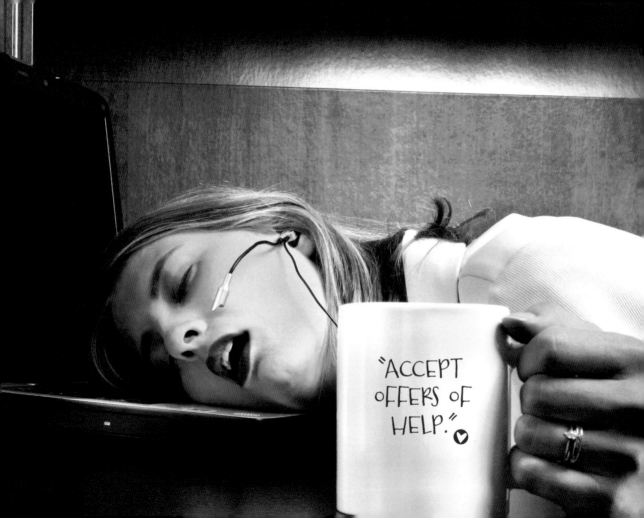

TAKE IT EASY
FATIGUE

Fatigue is one of the most common and difficult side effects of chemo. It's usually worse at the beginning and end of a treatment cycle. Planning ahead and making conscious decisions about your activities and how you order your day will make a big difference in how you feel.

To help keep your fatigue at a minimum:
- Don't try to do it all
- Accept help with shopping, housework, cooking and driving
- Get plenty of sleep. If you have trouble sleeping, tell your doctor
- Set aside time each day to rest
- Limit your activities
- Consciously think about your priorities
- Ask your doctor about exercise
- Eat a well-balanced diet
- Drink plenty of non-carbonated fluids
- Get up slowly from lying or sitting to prevent dizziness

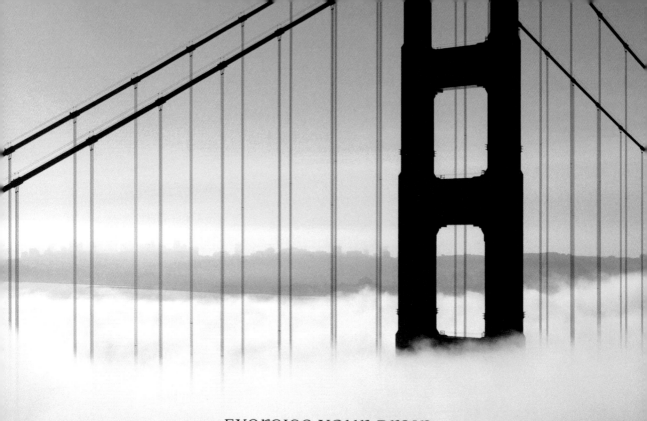

exercise your brain
to help lift the fog.

fogged in
chemo brain

Patients with "chemo brain" typically describe it like being in a mental fog. This includes memory lapses, trouble concentrating, being unable to remember details, the inability to multi-task and difficulty remembering common words. This **WILL** go away. To help manage it, try the following:

- Rest often and get plenty of sleep
- Exercise as much as you are able
- Get a weekly pill dispenser so you don't get meds mixed up
- Use a daily planner
- Establish routines
- Don't try to multi-task—focus on one thing at a time
- Exercise your brain with puzzles, Sudoku or by learning a new language
- Tell people so they will understand
- Call your most forgetful friend or relative and swap stories!

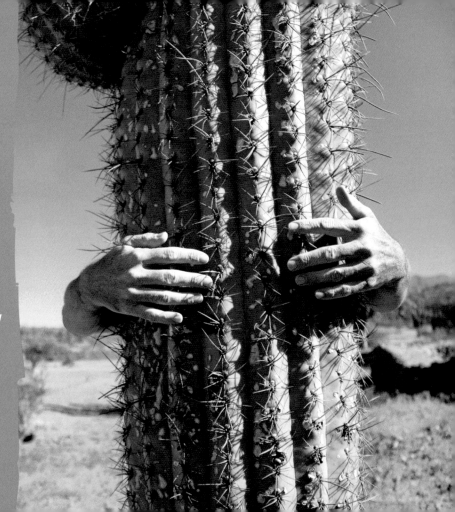

Don't Hide it!

Take pain seriously. If your regimen is not working, talk to your doctor and nurses. They can help you change it or refer you to a pain specialist who can. Talk to your family and close friends about how you're feeling, too. This will help them understand how they can help.

Ouch!
Pain

Some of the side effects you may experience with chemo are associated with pain. These include joint and muscle aches, headaches, burning and tingling in your hands and feet and stomach pain. Your pain could also be from the cancer itself and your doctor can prescribe medication to help ease your discomfort.

If you have pain all of the time, take your medication regularly and on time. If you skip doses and the pain gets severe, it will be much more difficult to control. If your pain is mild or occasional, you may only need to take the medication later in the day or before bed.

Pain management can also be helped through:
- Deep breathing exercises
- Yoga
- Massage
- Reflexology
- Acupuncture

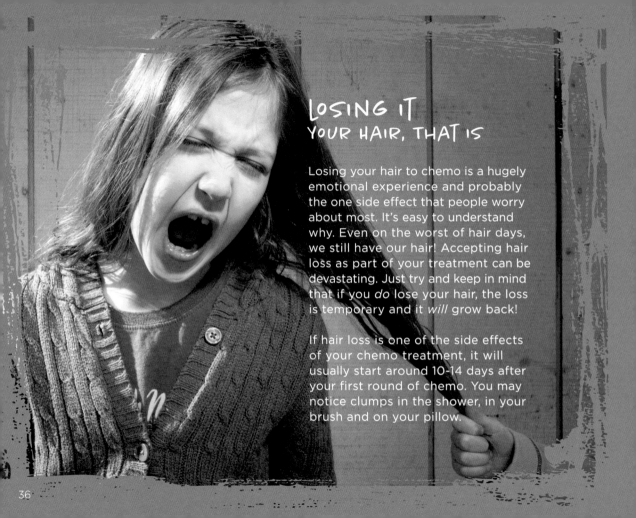

LOSING IT
YOUR HAIR, THAT IS

Losing your hair to chemo is a hugely emotional experience and probably the one side effect that people worry about most. It's easy to understand why. Even on the worst of hair days, we still have our hair! Accepting hair loss as part of your treatment can be devastating. Just try and keep in mind that if you *do* lose your hair, the loss is temporary and it *will* grow back!

If hair loss is one of the side effects of your chemo treatment, it will usually start around 10-14 days after your first round of chemo. You may notice clumps in the shower, in your brush and on your pillow.

Coping with the Loss

Some people find it helpful to cut their hair VERY short—about one inch all over. This is easier to handle than losing long clumps of hair. When the shorter hair starts getting too patchy, just shave it all off. Believe it or not, this looks and feels a lot better than you might think! If you do decide to shave your head, be sure to have a friend at your side who will not only support you but will make you laugh.

When your hair starts growing back, don't be surprised if the color and texture are different. Who knows, you just might get the curls you always dreamed of! Keep in mind that as it grows in, it may be fragile at first, so follow these simple guidelines:

- Use baby hair products
- Avoid using a hair dryer
- Don't use any heated styling tools

"WHEN YOUR HAIR STARTS FALLING OUT, DON'T TRY TO PULL IT OUT - THAT WILL HURT! JUST CUT IT OFF." ♥

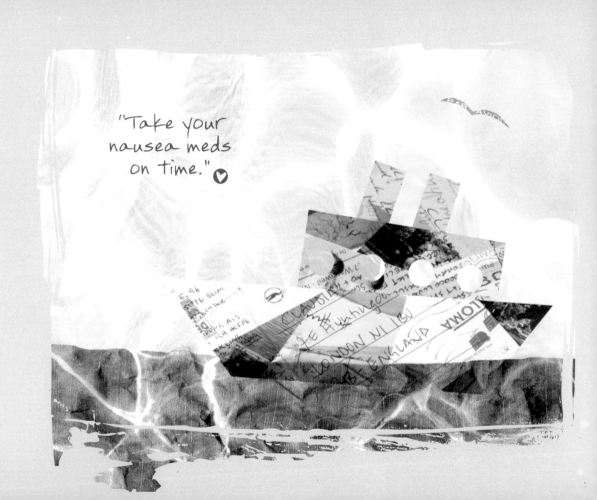

"Take your
nausea meds
on time."

Keep it Down
Nausea and Vomiting

Most chemo patients get nauseated, and may throw up. Many drugs are available to prevent and treat nausea and vomiting, so call your doctor and find the one that may work for you. You should also try the following:

- Wear loose-fitting clothes
- Don't go to chemo on an empty stomach
- Eat small, frequent meals
- Stay away from sweet, fried and fatty foods
- Eat cold or room-temperature foods, they have fewer strong smells
- Chew your food well
- Eat and drink slowly
- Drink liquids an hour before and after meals—not with meals
- Drink cool, non-carbonated liquids
- Suck on ice cubes and regular or ginger mints
- Refrain from lying down for two hours after eating
- Keep in mind that although it may not feel like it, this *will* pass

on the run
intestinal problems

During chemo, good cells in your body, like those in the intestinal lining, are destroyed—and that can lead to diarrhea and constipation.

Frequent diarrhea causes dehydration and weight loss. It's disruptive to your daily activities and adds to your fatigue. Your doctor can order medication for you if this becomes a problem.

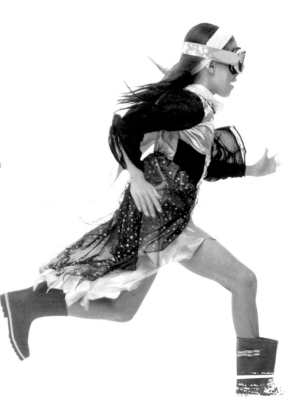

To help avoid diarrhea or ease the discomfort:

- Eat small amounts frequently
- Avoid coffee, tea, sweets and dairy products
- Avoid high-fiber foods
- Increase your amount of low-fiber foods
- Follow the BRAT diet—bananas, white rice, applesauce, toast—as a start
- Avoid fried, greasy and fatty foods and carbonated drinks
- Eat foods rich in potassium such as bananas, oranges, potatoes, peaches and apricots
- Eat foods high in protein
- Drink plenty of fluids
- Try Imodium®, Pepto-Bismol™ or Kaopectate®—these can be purchased over the counter
- Use Desitin® or A+D® Ointment around the anal area if the skin starts breaking down
- Call your doctor if you have diarrhea 4-5 times in a day and the above suggestions aren't helping

Constipation is also a challenge because it can cause abdominal pain and bloating, which affects your appetite and ability to eat. Prevention is important here, as is early treatment.

To prevent and treat this problem:

- Drink plenty of fluids, 8-10 glasses a day. Warm fluids are especially helpful
- Eat high-fiber foods such as fresh fruits and vegetables, prunes, raisins, nuts and bran
- Add bran to your diet gradually as too much can cause diarrhea. Start with 2 teaspoons a day sprinkled on food and gradually increase to 4-6 teaspoons
- Get some exercise
- Try Colace® capsules with Metamucil®
- Call your doctor if you haven't had a bowel movement in three days

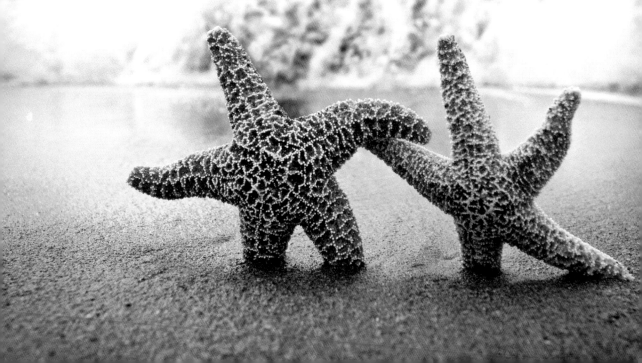

A friend is a present you give yourself. Call that friend you can share anything with.

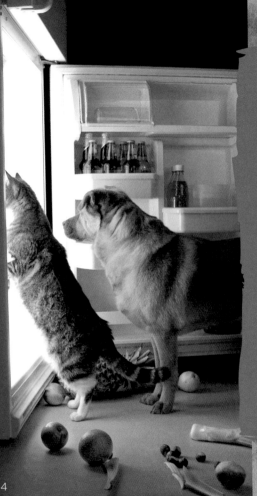

CULINARY CHALLENGE
CHANGES IN APPETITE

In one way or another, your appetite will probably be affected by chemo, so it's important to plan ahead and be creative in finding foods that you enjoy eating.

You may not be able to eat due to nausea, sores in your mouth, depression and/or fatigue. Chemo also causes food to taste differently—sometimes it's too sweet or too bitter, and it may leave a metallic taste in your mouth. Some people even temporarily lose their sense of taste, which also makes eating difficult.

To help ease your changing appetite:
- Take a walk before meals
- Rinse your mouth out before meals
- Eat smaller, more frequent meals and snacks
- Make sure to eat plenty of protein
- Try new foods and recipes
- Change your routine by trying new places to eat
- Avoid concentrated sweet or sour foods
- Dilute sweet beverages with water
- Use plastic spoons, knives and forks if a metallic taste becomes a problem
- Call friends and family and ask them to bring over their favorite dish—try each one!

"DON'T EAT YOUR FAVORITE FOODS WHEN YOU DON'T FEEL GOOD BECAUSE YOU'LL NEVER WANT THEM AGAIN WHEN CHEMO IS OVER."

BACK UP!!
GO BACK TO DENTAL CARE. THOSE TIPS WILL ALSO HELP PREVENT MOUTH SORES.

INSIDE OUT
Sore mouth, Gums & throat

Mouth sores are common during chemo and can affect your nutrition and cause pain if they get severe. Plan ahead and be ready, using the following tips:

- Apply cold-sore medication on sores *immediately* after they develop
- Use Cool Mint Chloraseptic® Sore Throat Spray
- Rinse with a solution of 1 cup water, 1 teaspoon baking soda and 1 teaspoon salt. Do this after meals and before bedtime. Increase this to every 2 hours while awake if necessary
- Drink plenty of liquids *using a straw* to bypass the sores
- Eat cold or room-temperature foods
- Eat soft foods such as scrambled eggs, mashed potatoes, yogurt, pudding, milk shakes, cooked cereal and soups
- Dip hard food in liquid or blend your food if necessary
- Avoid acidic, salty, spicy, rough, coarse and dry foods
- Suck on ice, popsicles or sugarless hard candy
- If you smoke—STOP!

Note: Use BIOTENE® mouth spray or other BIOTENE® brand products

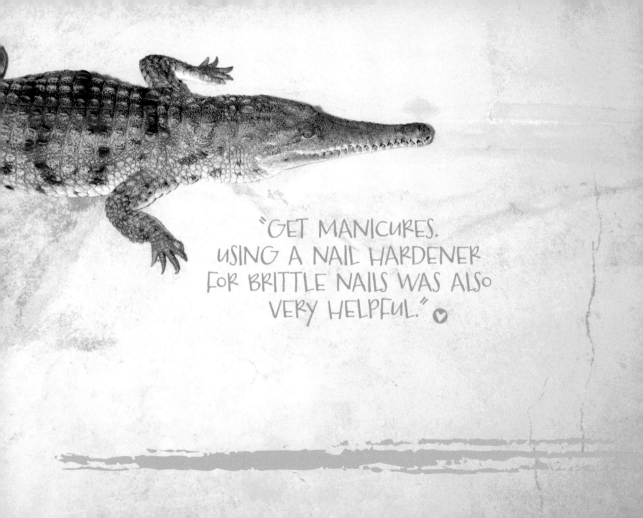

"GET MANICURES.
USING A NAIL HARDENER
FOR BRITTLE NAILS WAS ALSO
VERY HELPFUL."

SCALES TO NAILS
SKIN AND NAIL PROBLEMS

It's not unusual to have skin problems such as redness, itching, acne, dryness or peeling during chemo treatments. Blistering and peeling of the hands and feet are also common. This can be prevented by avoiding heat or friction to the hands and feet the day before and three days after a treatment.

You may also notice a dark line up the vein where you get chemo. Don't worry—this will eventually go away. Your skin may be more sensitive to the sun than ever before, so make sure you use sun protection. Nails may become brittle and break more easily.

To treat these conditions:

- Keep your face clean and dry
- Apply cornstarch to itchy skin
- Take shorter, warm showers instead of longer, hot ones and apply lotion or oil while your skin is still damp
- Use moisturizers on your face as well as a deeply hydrating mask
- Avoid perfume and cologne as they contain alcohol, which is drying
- Use sunscreen and wear long sleeves, pants and a hat when outdoors
- Get manicures and pedicures regularly, selecting a salon with high sanitation standards to prevent infection
- Prevent blisters on your feet with well-fitting shoes
- Wear socks or shoes at all times to protect the tender skin of your feet

"I MADE THE MISTAKE OF CUTTING MY NAILS TOO SHORT. NOTHING ON MY BODY IS GROWING AND NOW MY FINGERTIPS ARE SORE."

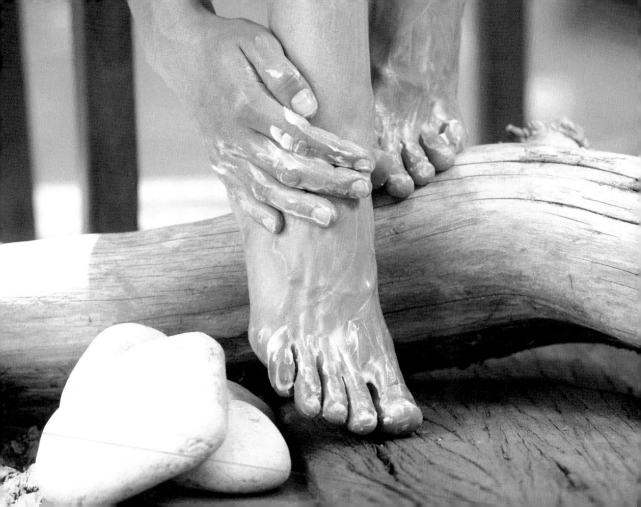

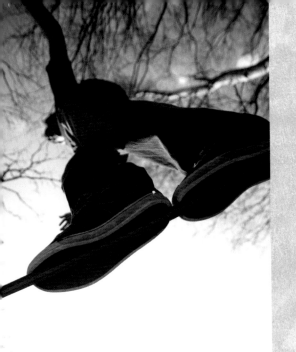

Nice n' Easy
Nerve and Muscle Problems

Certain chemo drugs can cause a peripheral neuropathy, which is a dysfunction of the small nerves throughout the body. It is most common in hands and feet and is similar to the difficulties experienced by diabetics, the difference being that with chemo it's usually temporary.

Tell your doctor if you experience any of the following symptoms:

- Tingling/burning sensations
- Weakness/numbness in hands and feet
- Loss of balance
- Clumsiness
- Difficulty picking up objects
- Trouble buttoning clothes
- Difficulty walking
- Jaw pain
- Hearing loss
- Vision changes
- Stomach pain
- Constipation

It's important to take precautions to protect yourself from injury if these symptoms occur. You should always:

- Be careful with sharp instruments such as scissors, knives and razors
- Move slowly and carefully
- Hold on to handrails
- Use a bath mat in the shower or tub
- Remove things from the floor that you might trip over
- Secure area rugs
- Wear well-fitting rubber-soled shoes

"COLD COMPRESSES WORK WELL FOR ITCHY EYES. SOAK A WASHCLOTH IN ICE WATER." ♥

LOOKIN' GOOD
EYE AND VISION CHANGES

Chemo affects your eyes, just as it does the rest of your body. Because the chemo drugs pass through your tear ducts, they can cause such common problems as:

- Dry eye syndrome—when the ducts become clogged
- Watery, itchy eyes
- Conjunctivitis—redness and inflammation

You can treat these conditions with lubricating eye drops and ice packs. If you wear contact lenses and develop any of these conditions, you may be more comfortable with glasses. Just be sure your prescription is up to date.

Chemo can also cause sensitivity to bright light and sudden changes in light, a condition known as photophobia. A great-looking pair of sunglasses should do the trick, but if your symptoms are severe, have your oncologist refer you to an ophthalmologist.

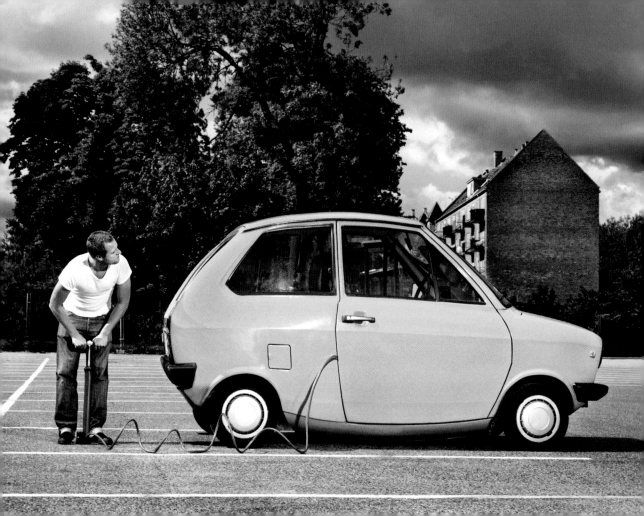

UP, UP AND AWAY
FLUID RETENTION

Chemo and hormonal changes often cause fluid retention. This fluid tends to build up in your hands, feet, face and stomach and can make you feel puffy and uncomfortable. It can also build up around your heart and lungs, making it more difficult to breathe, causing you to cough and possibly have an irregular heartbeat. These are all symptoms that you should tell your doctor about because you may need medication to control them.

To help monitor your water retention:

- Weigh yourself at the same time each day using the same scale. This will help your doctor evaluate how much your fluid levels fluctuate
- Your doctor may ask you to limit your salt intake and the amount of liquids you drink during this time

Write down your daily weight and remember to take the log to your doctor's appointment.

"DRINK
LOTS OF
WATER!"

JUST ADD WATER
KIDNEY AND BLADDER IRRITATION

Chemo drugs can irritate your bladder and may cause damage to your kidneys. This happens because chemo drugs are eliminated from the body in your urine and are concentrated there. Drinking plenty of fluids helps dilute the chemo drugs and makes them less toxic as they exit your body. Your urine may turn an orange, red or yellow color, or take on a strong medicinal odor. This is normal and not something to be concerned about.

*However, you **should** call your doctor if you experience any of the following:*

- Pain or burning during urination
- Frequent urination
- Feeling that you can't get to the bathroom fast enough to urinate
- Bloody urine
- Fever
- Chills

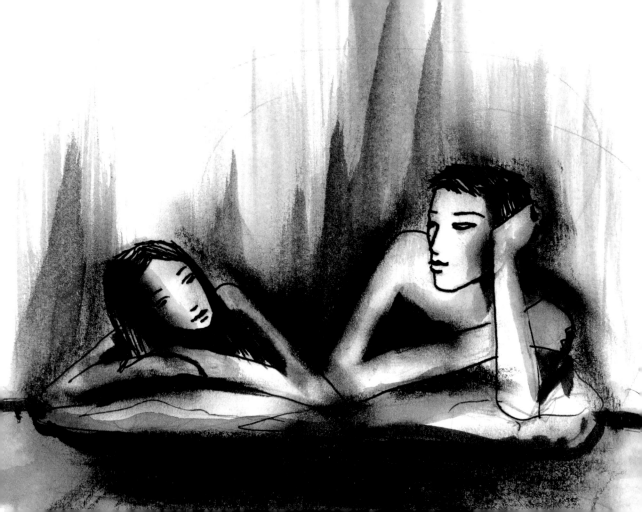

Stay in Touch
Sex and Reproduction

Sexual changes are not uncommon during chemo. Whether you have difficulty with this will depend on the type of chemo drugs you're taking, your age and other illnesses you may have.

What can happen? Because chemo can damage ovaries, women may experience changes in hormone levels leading to menopause-like symptoms, including hot flashes, vaginal dryness or itching, irregular or no menstrual periods as well as bladder or vaginal infections.

To manage these symptoms:
- Dress in layers that you can remove during a hot flash
- Be active and exercise as much as possible
- Avoid wearing tight pants
- Wear cotton underwear or underwear with a cotton lining
- Use a water-based vaginal lubricant during sexual intercourse

Both men and women may find that they're unable to climax due to changes in the blood flow to sexual organs. Men may also experience impotency during chemo due to hormonal changes. It's important to use a condom during sex as there may be small amounts of chemo in the semen that you don't want passed on to your partner.

Birth control is essential for men and women who are undergoing chemo. That's because the chemo drugs go directly from the mother to the fetus or from the father to the fetus during intercourse. Exposure to chemo can be very harmful for a developing fetus, especially during the first trimester. If your partner *does* become pregnant while you're undergoing chemo, you should continue to use condoms.

Infertility is also a possible side effect for both sexes. This is because chemo can damage the ovaries, leading to fewer healthy eggs and it can cause sperm to be less potent. These effects can be permanent, so be sure to talk to your doctor before starting chemo if you plan to have children.

If you or your partner has sexual or reproductive health concerns, be sure to talk to your oncologist about them and consider a referral to a health care provider who specializes in reproductive issues.

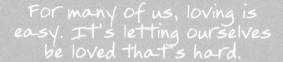

For many of us, loving is easy. It's letting ourselves be loved that's hard.

Sex is one way to express your love. Here are some others:

- Watch the sun rise together
- Give each other a massage
- Look deeply into each other's eyes
- Reminisce about the "firsts" in your relationship
- Read aloud to each other
- Fall asleep in each other's arms
- Take your partner's "to do" list and do it for them
- Tell your partner why they're beautiful
- Thank your partner for something they've done
- Share your hopes and fears

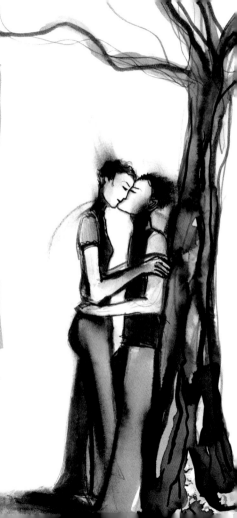

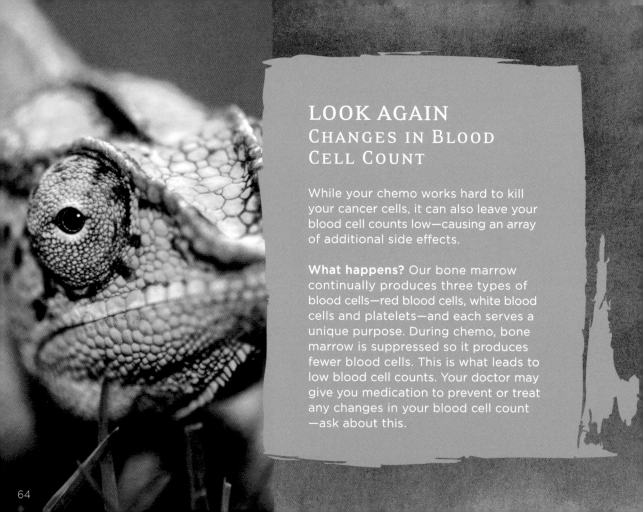

LOOK AGAIN
CHANGES IN BLOOD CELL COUNT

While your chemo works hard to kill your cancer cells, it can also leave your blood cell counts low—causing an array of additional side effects.

What happens? Our bone marrow continually produces three types of blood cells—red blood cells, white blood cells and platelets—and each serves a unique purpose. During chemo, bone marrow is suppressed so it produces fewer blood cells. This is what leads to low blood cell counts. Your doctor may give you medication to prevent or treat any changes in your blood cell count —ask about this.

Red blood cells carry oxygen in your blood. If they are low, your heart will have to work harder to get enough oxygen to your body. This, in turn, may cause:

- Fatigue
- Dizziness
- Weakness
- Pounding or fast heart rate
- Shortness of breath
- Pale skin
- Feeling cold

White blood cells are the army that fights infection. A decrease in these cells makes it more difficult for your body to fight bacteria that cause infections. If this number drops too low, your chemo may be delayed or your medication adjusted.

IF YOU THINK YOU HAVE AN INFECTION, CALL YOUR DOCTOR IMMEDIATELY TO START TREATMENT.

Signs of infection to look for:
- Fever of more than 100.5° F
- Chills and/or sweating
- Diarrhea or abdominal pain
- Burning during urination
- Unusual vaginal discharge
- Severe cough or sore throat
- Itching, redness, pus, swelling or tenderness around a wound, sore or catheter site

To help prevent infections:
- Wash your hands frequently and carry a hand sanitizer
- Ask friends not to visit when they are sick
- Avoid crowds
- Don't bite, tear or cut your cuticles
- Use an electric razor while shaving to avoid cuts from a razor blade
- Use lotions and oils to prevent cracking skin due to dryness
- Use antiseptic ointment on cuts
- Wear protective gloves when gardening or washing the dishes
- Be careful around animals and do NOT clean up their waste
- Wash raw vegetables and fruits before eating
- Do not eat raw or undercooked seafood, meat, poultry or eggs
- Always wear shoes or slippers

Platelets make your blood clot to stop bleeding. A decrease in the number of these cells may cause easy bleeding or bruising. Many over-the-counter drugs like aspirin or ibuprofen will increase bleeding by affecting how platelets work. Many herbs and supplements also increase bleeding, so make sure to tell your doctor *everything* you are taking and ask what medicines you should take for pain management. Acetaminophen is generally a safe option.

Report any of the following symptoms to your doctor:
- Unexpected bruising
- Small red dots under your skin
- Red or pink urine
- Black or bloody bowel movements
- Bleeding from the gums or nose
- Bad headaches
- Muscle and/or joint pain

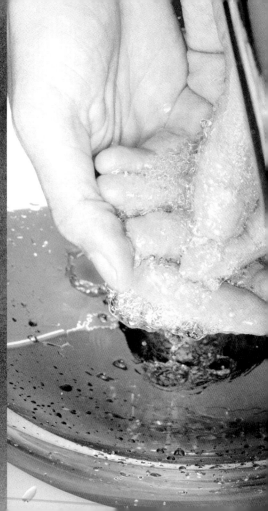

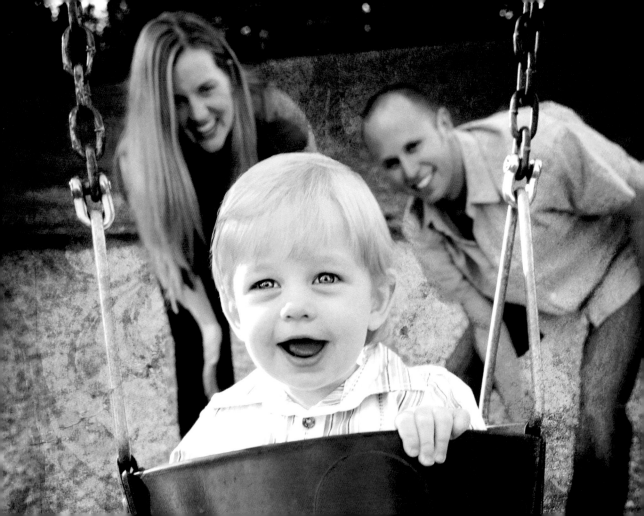

constant companion
A natural HIGH!

NO ONE EVER REGRETS THE TIME THEY'VE SPENT LAUGHING.

LAUGHTER
The Best Medicine 71

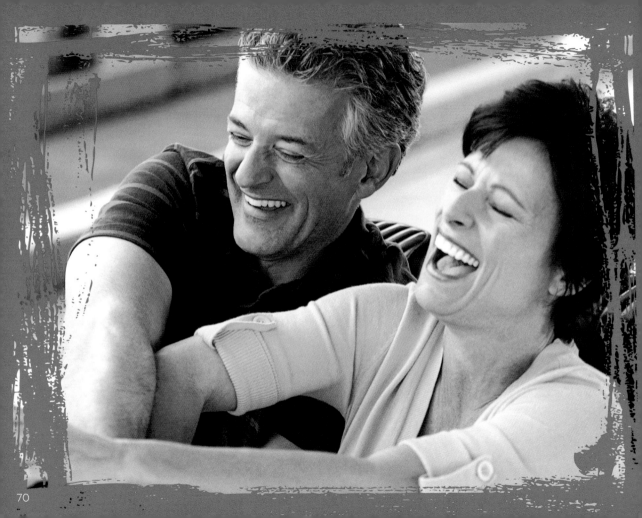

LAUGHTER
THE BEST MEDICINE

Go ahead, laugh. It's really ok! It may do more good than you realize.

Modern research into the healing properties of laughter began in the 1970s when Norman Cousins reported on how he checked himself out of a hospital and into a hotel to watch funny movies. The more he laughed, the better he felt, until he finally overcame a painful and debilitating condition.

There is now an abundance of research and literature on the benefits of laughter:

- It decreases the level of stress hormones in the body
- It increases the antibodies that fight infection, thus strengthening the immune system
- Another *major benefit* of laughter is the increase in endorphins, the body's natural pain killers, which are even more powerful than morphine

Hospitals have begun to offer laughter therapy to their patients, and organizations have started laughter clubs. These are all for the purpose of enhancing wellness and healing. Humor has even been shown to change negative emotions like anger, anxiety and depression. Unfortunately, humor generally leaves you precisely when you need it most.

It is important to learn to laugh at yourself. When we laugh at ourselves, our difficulties become much easier to bear and those around us also relax. They are given permission to ask how we're doing and to talk about it.

So don't be afraid to laugh. Go watch that comedy or read that funny book. Seek out your funniest friends and laugh until your belly hurts. You may mix tears with your laughter but you will feel better and heal better for it.

Laughter truly *is* the best medicine.

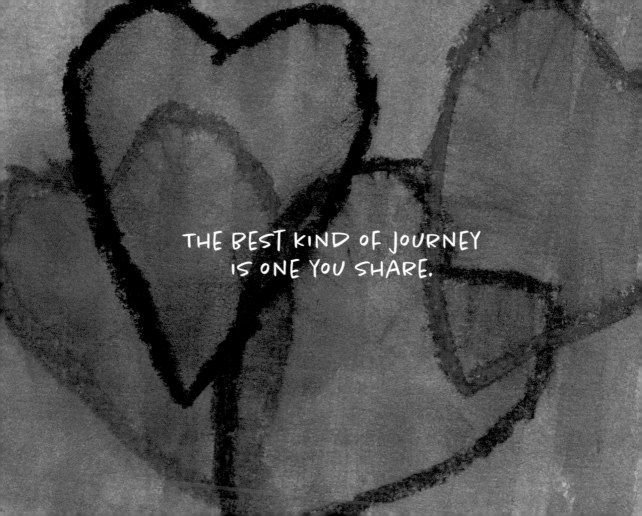

THE BEST KIND OF JOURNEY
IS ONE YOU SHARE.

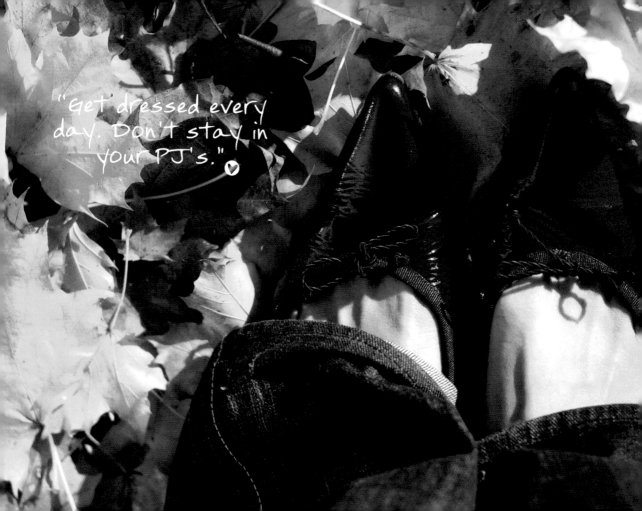

"Get dressed every day. Don't stay in your PJ's." ♥

TRAVEL TIPS
QUOTES FROM CHEMO GRADUATES

"Have a built-in rest period EVERY DAY, and don't overdo it on days you feel good or you will pay later."

"You need a barf bucket. I never used mine, but you should have one—just in case."

"Take your nausea meds on time and don't miss any of them, even if you think you don't need them."

"Get a weekly pill dispenser so you don't get your meds mixed up."

"Everyone needs a blanket for chemo. Those places are always cold."

"Everyone I know got constipated— no diarrhea."

"I documented my stages of hair loss and growth in photos. Not everyone can do that."

"You may be tired enough that you'll want to get a handicap parking placard for awhile. AAA members can get them at the AAA office, and they are available from the DMV (but the lines are longer). Your doctor will need to fill out a form for you to get one."

"My face feels like I've had a chemical peel. I'm hoping my skin will look better when I'm done."

"My oncologist believes in the therapeutic effects of massage and reflexology. I had one every evening before my next chemo session."

"PRIORITIZE."

"If you lose your eyelashes or brows, use eyeliner to line your eyes then smudge it so it doesn't look so harsh. Sketch on eyebrows lightly and smudge a little."

"Peppermint and ginger teas help nausea."

"It's helpful to have a "worry rock" to keep your hands busy when you are stressed."

"Any noise during chemo really bothered me—even music sometimes. I just wanted it quiet."

"My "chemo brain" was so bad that I couldn't even read or watch TV. The only thing I could do was talk to my friends."

"A mini handheld fan is good for hot flashes."

"Yoga was really helpful for me to relax and focus on the rest of my life."

"Practice deep-breathing exercises."

"Don't forget to call your best friend."

VISIT US ONLINE AT:
www.chemocompanioncares.com

entourage
ACKNOWLEDGMENTS

The greatest of thanks goes to:

❥ Those who opened their hearts to relive their experiences—Audrey Benson, Nancy Turk, Jennifer Sheppard, and my sister, Kaye Whitney.

❥ Those who shared stories and tips from their patients, families and friends— Sheri Naragon, Janice Smith, Gail Walters and Katharine Walters.

❥ Those who offered professional advice and reviewed the manuscript— Dr. Charles Goodacre, *Dean of the School of Dentistry at Loma Linda University,* Dr. Dennis Hilliard, *oncologist in Redlands, California,* Susan Troy and Desiree Kumar, *oncology nurse specialists.*

❥ Those who lent their support—Dr. Ben Carson and Elder Jerry Lutz.

❥ The two who pushed from behind—Tammy Stream and Dr. Linda Wat.

❥ The one who had the vision to share this book with others, whose constant determination and untiring campaigning carried this project to completion— Lanette Sprengel Mohr.

Jeanie

Connection is key! My deepest thanks go out to the following:

- God greatly blessed me with this project and I am humbly grateful.

- Kaye Whitney for your graceful inspiration and inviting me on your journey. Your miracles are many. Jeanie Sprengel, thank you for entrusting me with your dream. It has been a privilege collaborating with you and others in bringing this book to life. It is great being your partner.

- To the esteemed within the Cancer Community who extended themselves and offered enthusiastic support to our concept—especially Andy Miller with the *Lance Armstrong Foundation*, Diane Blum from *Cancer Care*, Hala Moddelmog, Diana Rowden and Susan Brown at *Susan G. Komen for the Cure*.

- To the group that helped us 'do the work' and do it right - Kristie Severn, Greg Shoemaker, Kara Wiley Flynn, Michelle Simmons, Martha Craig, Jim Becker, Chad Freeman and Ken Stream.

- To those who fill the blurry lines between family and friends, and friends-of-friends. For sharing your connections, your time, expertise and most of all—your love: Sunny & Tisha Vanderbeck, Fritzi Woods, Kevin Scott, Gary & Denise Yiatchos, Trina Seligman, Holly Pankratz, Gary & Jorie Gulbranson, Westminster Women, Roger and Joanne Mohr, Kathi Speller, Josh, Lexi, Parker and Selah Clayton, and to Scot Mohr, the perfect husband for me.

Lanette

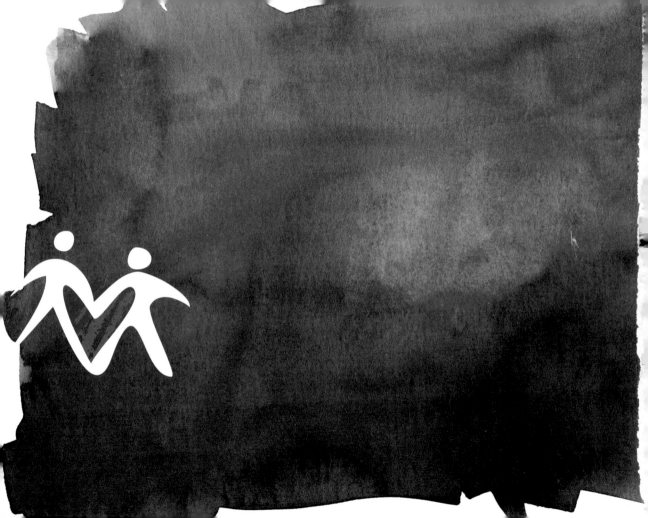